CHAIR YOGA

for

SENIORS OVER 60

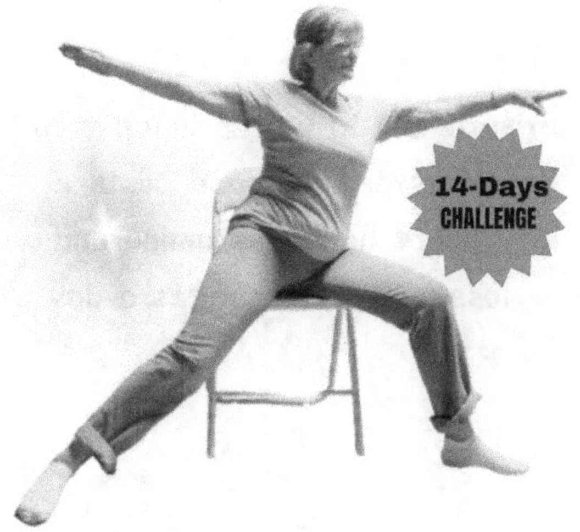

Matthew L. Moreno

CHAIR YOGA
FOR
SENIORS OVER 60

An ultimate step by step illustrated guide to master, for good posture, mobility, heart health, stamina and weight loss under 10 minutes a day

Matthew L.Moreno

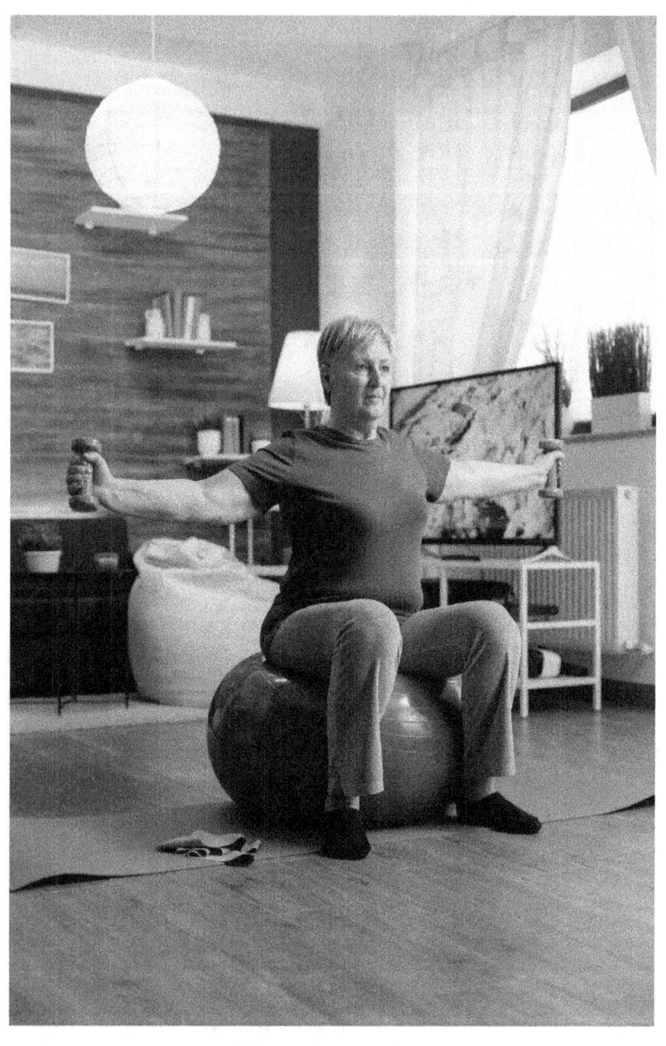

INTRODUCTION

In the bustling heart of a small town, an individual's life was forever transformed by the simple act of sitting in a chair. Meet Margaret. At 68, her days were marked by stiffness, aches, and the challenges that come with aging gracefully. Until one serendipitous day when she stumbled upon a chair yoga class at the local community center.

As she tentatively sank into the supportive cushion of her chair, little did Margaret know that this ordinary piece of furniture would become her gateway to extraordinary well-being. With every gentle stretch, every mindful breath, her body and spirit began to awaken. The stiffness that once plagued her movements melted away, replaced by a newfound ease. Chair yoga became more than a routine; it became her sanctuary, a source of resilience, and a catalyst for a life filled with vitality.

In today's fast-paced world, the quest for holistic well-being often seems like an uphill battle, especially for those in the golden years. Yet, nestled within the folds of a familiar chair lies an incredible secret: the transformative power of chair yoga. This ancient practice, adapted thoughtfully for seniors, offers a gateway to health, flexibility, and peace of mind—all from the comfort of a seated position.

Through a harmonious blend of gentle movements, breathwork, and mindfulness, chair yoga extends an inviting hand to individuals seeking to rejuvenate their bodies, calm their minds, and embrace the fullness of life. Whether you're an absolute beginner or someone seeking alternative ways to stay active, this book serves as your trusted companion on the journey to discovering the transformative magic of chair yoga.

Join me as we embark on a remarkable voyage—one where each chapter unfolds a tapestry of accessible poses, breathing exercises, and wellness insights tailored to empower and uplift seniors over 60.

Welcome to a world where chairs are not just for sitting; they're vehicles for transformation, healing, and a renewed zest for life.

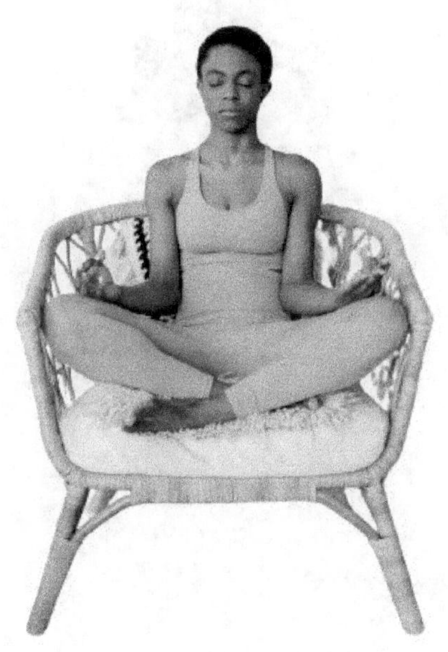

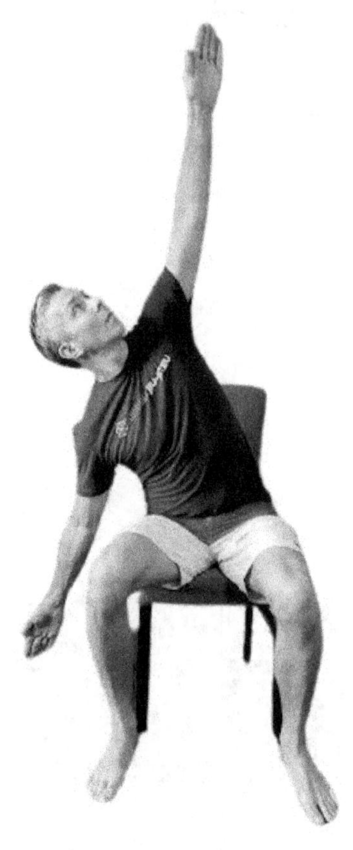

CHAPTER 1: CHAIR YOGA

What is yoga and it history

Yoga, an ancient practice dating back thousands of years, embodies a rich tapestry of tradition, spirituality, and holistic wellness. Its roots delve into the depths of ancient India, where it began as a philosophical and spiritual discipline.

The origins of yoga are intertwined with the Vedic civilization, around 5000 years ago. Its earliest traces can be found in the sacred texts of the Vedas, specifically in the Rigveda, where hymns suggest the contemplation of inner and outer realities, emphasizing a connection between the mind, body, and the universe.

The foundational text of yoga, the "Yoga Sutras," was compiled by the sage Patanjali around 400 CE. These sutras serve as a guiding light, outlining the principles and philosophy of yoga. Patanjali delineated the eight limbs of yoga, known as Ashtanga Yoga, which forms the bedrock of classical yoga philosophy. These limbs encompass ethical guidelines (Yamas and Niyamas), physical postures (Asanas), breath control (Pranayama), sense withdrawal (Pratyahara), concentration (Dharana), meditation (Dhyana), and enlightenment (Samadhi).

Throughout the centuries, yoga evolved, incorporating various schools of thought, practices, and techniques. Hatha Yoga emerged in the Middle Ages, focusing on physical postures (Asanas) and breath control (Pranayama) to prepare the body for meditation and spiritual growth.

The practice of yoga traversed continents, reaching the Western world in the late 19th and early 20th centuries. Indian yogis like Swami Vivekananda and later teachers such as Paramahansa Yogananda and B.K.S. Iyengar played pivotal roles in popularizing yoga globally. They introduced diverse yoga styles, emphasizing not only physical postures but also meditation, breathwork, and philosophy.

Today, yoga transcends borders and cultures, celebrated as a holistic practice that nurtures physical, mental, and spiritual well-being. Its profound impact on health, stress reduction, and inner harmony continues to resonate, inviting individuals worldwide to embark on a journey of self-discovery and inner transformation through this ancient, timeless practice.

Yoga principle and types

Yoga stands tall on a few guiding principles:
1. Unity: It's about bringing harmony between the mind, body, and spirit.
2. Breath: Focus on breathing to connect with the present moment and calm the mind.
3. Postures: These are physical poses (asanas) that enhance flexibility, strength, and balance.

4. **Meditation**: Practicing mindfulness to quiet the mind and find inner peace.

5. **Relaxation:** Allowing oneself to unwind and release tension through deep relaxation techniques.

Types of Yoga

1. **Hatha Yoga:** Gentle and foundational, focusing on basic poses and breathing exercises, suitable for beginners.

2. **Vinyasa Yoga:** A dynamic flow of movements synchronized with breath, offering a more energetic practice.

3. **Ashtanga Yoga:** A structured sequence of poses that demand strength, flexibility, and breath control.

4. **Kundalini Yoga:** Emphasizes the release of energy through breath work, chanting, and poses.

5. **Bikram Yoga:** Conducted in a heated room, consisting of a set series of 26 poses aimed at detoxification.

6. **Yin Yoga:** A slower-paced practice involving longer holds in poses to target

deep connective tissues and enhance flexibility.

7. Restorative Yoga: A soothing practice using props to support the body, promoting relaxation and healing.

8. Iyengar Yoga: Focuses on precision in alignment using props like blocks and straps to help perform poses with accuracy.

Each type offers its own flavor, catering to various needs—whether it's building strength, finding inner peace, or simply improving flexibility. Think of them like different paths leading to the same destination—a healthier, more balanced you.

These principles and types create a rich tapestry within the world of yoga, inviting everyone to explore and find the practice that resonates most with them.

What is Chair yoga ?

Chair yoga is like a gentle magic trick, transforming a simple chair into a haven of wellness. Picture this: instead of sprawling on a yoga mat, you're seated comfortably on a chair, exploring a world of movement, relaxation, and inner peace.

It's yoga's adaptable cousin, designed for everyone—regardless of age, flexibility, or physical limitations. This practice takes the ancient art of yoga and molds it to fit into the cozy space around your chair. From gentle stretches to graceful twists, it's a symphony of movements that embrace the support of your trusty seat.

The beauty of chair yoga lies in its simplicity. It's about harnessing the power of breath and movement while being seated, allowing you to experience the benefits of traditional yoga poses in a more accessible and manageable way.

Imagine reaching for the sky with a stretch while firmly rooted in your seat. Or gently turning your torso to release tension, all while feeling supported and secure. It's not just about the body; it's a mindful journey where your breath becomes a guiding companion, leading you into a state of calm and relaxation.

Chair yoga is a versatile ally. It caters to those with mobility issues, injuries, or anyone seeking a softer approach to yoga. It's a doorway to improved flexibility, reduced stress, and a more peaceful state of mind—all from the comfort of your chair.

This practice isn't confined to a specific place or time; it's portable, adaptable, and oh-so-inviting. Whether in an office, at home, or a community center, chair yoga invites you to embrace wellness wherever you are.

In essence, chair yoga is a gentle embrace, inviting you to explore the essence of yoga in a way that's kind, accessible, and profoundly beneficial. It's a reminder that the magic of yoga isn't limited by where you can stand or how far you can bend—it's a practice that meets you exactly where you are.

Benefits of chair yoga

Chair yoga is a beautiful gateway to well-being, offering a world of benefits in the simplest, most accessible ways. Imagine a practice that gently embraces you, regardless of age or physical ability, guiding you toward a healthier, more vibrant life.

Firstly, it's all about flexibility. With chair yoga, you get to stretch and move your body without the need to bend or twist on the floor. Those simple seated stretches and movements help loosen up stiff muscles, easing tension, and improving flexibility.

Then, there's strength. Believe it or not, sitting in a chair can help you build strength! Through various poses and movements, chair yoga works muscles you might not even realize you have. It's like a gentle workout that keeps your body strong and balanced.

Breath by breath, chair yoga teaches you the power of mindful breathing. It's not just about the poses; it's about syncing your movements with your breath. Learning to breathe deeply and calmly can reduce stress, calm your mind, and boost your energy levels.

One of the most wonderful benefits is how it helps with pain relief. Whether it's joint pain, backache, or discomfort from sitting too long, chair yoga offers gentle movements that can ease those aches and pains. It's like a soothing balm for your body.

And let's not forget about relaxation. Chair yoga creates a space for peace and tranquility, even in the midst of a busy day. As you practice, you'll find yourself unwinding, letting go of stress, and inviting calmness into your life.

Importantly, chair yoga is inclusive. It doesn't matter if you're an experienced yogi or a complete beginner, or if you have limited mobility. It welcomes everyone, meeting you right where you are and supporting your journey towards better health.

In these simple movements, seated poses, and mindful breaths lies a treasure trove of benefits. Chair yoga isn't just about the body; it's a holistic embrace that nurtures your mind, body, and spirit, inviting you to discover a path to wellness that's gentle, accessible, and oh-so-rewarding.

CHAPTER 2: PREPARING FOR CHAIR YOGA

Building the Right Mind

This book doesn't just focus on the physical practice; it delves into nurturing the right mindset for chair yoga. It explores the importance of cultivating a positive attitude, patience, and self-compassion. Through gentle encouragement and mindfulness exercises, it guides seniors toward embracing the practice with a mindset of openness and acceptance. It emphasizes that the journey of chair yoga starts within, fostering mental resilience and a sense of peace.

Overcoming Common Obstacles to Starting Yoga

Starting something new can be daunting, especially for seniors venturing into yoga.

This book addresses common concerns such as fear of injury, self-doubt, or feeling intimidated. It provides relatable stories, practical advice, and testimonials from seniors who overcame similar obstacles. It offers gentle encouragement, explaining how chair yoga is tailored for their needs, making it accessible and safe, thereby instilling confidence in the reader to begin their yoga journey.

Tips for Practicing Chair Yoga Safely

Safety is paramount, especially for seniors. This book meticulously outlines safety guidelines, from choosing the right chair to explaining proper posture and alignment during poses. It offers modifications for different abilities and health conditions, empowering seniors to practice with confidence. Additionally, it highlights the importance of listening to one's body, taking breaks, and seeking professional guidance if needed.

Things to Avoid

In understanding the nuances of chair yoga, the book educates readers about practices or movements that might not be suitable or safe for seniors. It provides clear instructions on what to avoid, emphasizing the importance of gentle, controlled movements to prevent strain or injury. By highlighting these precautions, the book ensures a safer and more enjoyable yoga experience.

Creating Chair Yoga Practice at Home

For seniors seeking the comfort and convenience of practicing at home, this book serves as a guide. It outlines step-by-step instructions on creating a conducive space, selecting appropriate props, and designing a personalized chair yoga routine. It encourages consistency, offering tips to stay motivated and dedicated to their practice.

Each aspect of the book "Chair Yoga for Seniors Over 60" is carefully crafted to support seniors in not just practicing yoga but embracing it as a holistic lifestyle choice for their well-being.

CHAPTER 3: BREATHING AND WARM-UP EXERCISES

Chair Yoga Breathing Exercises
Embracing Serenity Through Breath

In the world of chair yoga, the breath becomes a bridge between the physical body and the mind, fostering a sense of tranquility and inner harmony. Breathing exercises, known as pranayama, are a cornerstone of this practice, offering a pathway to relaxation, heightened awareness, and overall well-being.

The process of chair yoga breathing exercises begins with finding a comfortable seated position. Seniors, often the practitioners of chair yoga, are encouraged to sit tall yet relaxed on a sturdy chair, ensuring their feet are firmly grounded on the floor and their spine is comfortably aligned.

The journey into the realm of breath awareness starts with mindfulness. The instructor guides participants through gentle reminders to bring attention to their breath. They're encouraged to notice the natural rhythm of their inhalations and exhalations, without attempting to change or control it initially.

The exercises progress gradually, often beginning with simple techniques like Deep Abdominal Breathing or Belly Breathing. This foundational practice involves inhaling deeply through the nose, allowing the belly to expand fully, and then exhaling slowly through pursed lips, gently contracting the abdominal muscles. This technique helps seniors to connect with their diaphragmatic breathing, which promotes relaxation and reduces stress.

As practitioners grow accustomed to this foundational practice, they advance to more nuanced techniques. Alternate Nostril Breathing, or Nadi Shodhana, is a popular technique introduced in chair yoga. This method involves using the thumb and ring finger to alternately close and open the nostrils while breathing. It aims to balance the left and right hemispheres of the brain, enhancing mental clarity and focus.

Chair yoga also introduces techniques like Box Breathing or Equal Breathing, where the inhalation, retention, exhalation, and pause between breaths are all of equal lengths. This pattern induces a sense of calmness and equilibrium within the body and mind.

Guidance is key in these exercises. The instructor's gentle cues and calming voice serve as beacons, guiding practitioners through each breath cycle. They emphasize the importance of patience and self-compassion, encouraging participants to honor their body's capabilities and never force or strain during the practice.

What makes chair yoga breathing exercises especially accessible and beneficial for seniors is their adaptability. The exercises can be modified to accommodate various mobility levels and health conditions. Sitting comfortably in a chair, participants can enjoy the benefits of breathwork without the need for complex physical postures.

As the session draws to a close, practitioners are invited to savor a few moments of stillness, basking in the afterglow of the breathing exercises. The gentle return to normal breathing patterns leaves them feeling rejuvenated, centered, and more at ease.

In essence, chair yoga breathing exercises are a gateway to inner peace and vitality. Through gentle, purposeful breathwork, seniors find a sanctuary within the rhythm of their breath—a sanctuary that nurtures their well-being, calms their mind, and fosters a deeper connection to the present moment.

This note offers an in-depth exploration of chair yoga breathing exercises, focusing on their gentle approach and benefits for practitioners.

Chair yoga warm-up and stretch exercises

Setting the Stage:
Before diving into warm-up and stretch exercises, finding a calm, quiet space with a sturdy chair is essential. Ensuring the chair is placed on a stable surface and is comfortable for seated movements is key. Comfortable clothing that allows free movement is recommended.

Mindful Breathing:
The session typically begins with a focus on mindful breathing. Seated comfortably, practitioners are guided to close their eyes, inhaling deeply through the nose and exhaling gently through the mouth. This helps center the mind, relax the body, and initiate a connection between breath and movement.

Gentle Warm-Up:

The warm-up phase starts gradually, involving gentle movements to awaken the body. This might include shoulder rolls, neck stretches, and gentle twists while seated on the chair. These movements aim to increase blood flow, loosen stiff muscles, and enhance flexibility without exerting strain.

Seated Stretches:
Moving into stretching exercises, practitioners are guided through a series of seated stretches. These encompass a range of motions targeting various muscle groups—hamstrings, hips, arms, and back. Each stretch is approached slowly and mindfully, respecting the body's limits and avoiding any discomfort.

Incorporating Breath:
Throughout the warm-up and stretch exercises, emphasis is placed on synchronizing movements with breath. Inhaling during the lengthening or opening phase of a stretch and exhaling during relaxation or release helps deepen the stretch and promotes relaxation.

Mindfulness and Awareness:
At the core of these exercises lies mindfulness and body awareness. Practitioners are encouraged to tune into their bodies, noticing sensations and respecting any limitations. Gentle reminders to avoid overstretching or pushing beyond comfort help maintain a safe practice.

Cool Down and Relaxation:
Following the stretching phase, a cool-down period ensues. This involves gentle movements to gradually bring the body back to a state of relaxation, such as slow neck rotations or gentle shoulder shrugs. The session often concludes with a guided relaxation or meditation, allowing practitioners to bask in the benefits of their practice.

Reflecting and Closing:
As the session draws to a close, practitioners are invited to reflect on the experience, acknowledging any changes in their body or mindset. A closing moment of

gratitude for the practice seals the session on a positive note.

Chair yoga warm-up and stretch exercises, conducted with mindfulness and care, serve as a gentle yet impactful journey towards enhancing flexibility, promoting relaxation, and nurturing overall well-being. This thoughtful approach ensures a safe, accessible, and fulfilling practice for individuals of all ages and abilities.

CHAPTER 4: 14 DAYS BEGINNER CHAIR YOGA CHALLENGE

FOCUS ON POSTURE

Day 1: *Seated Mountain Pose*

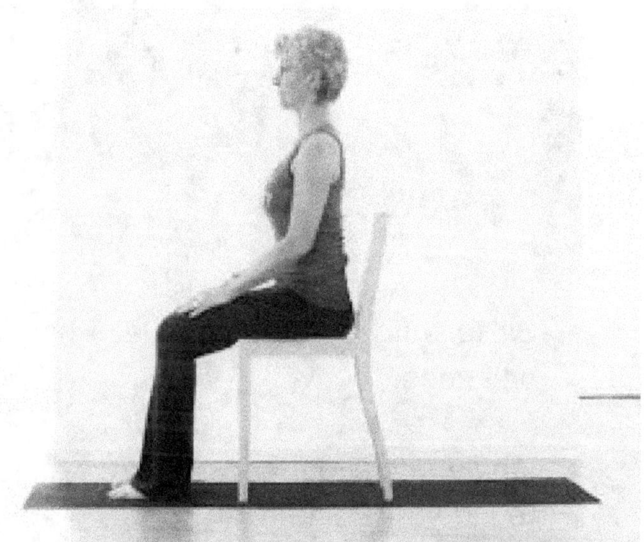

- Sit tall in your chair, feet flat on the ground.

- Roll shoulders back, elongate the spine, and engage core muscles.

Day 2: *Seated Cat-Cow Stretch*

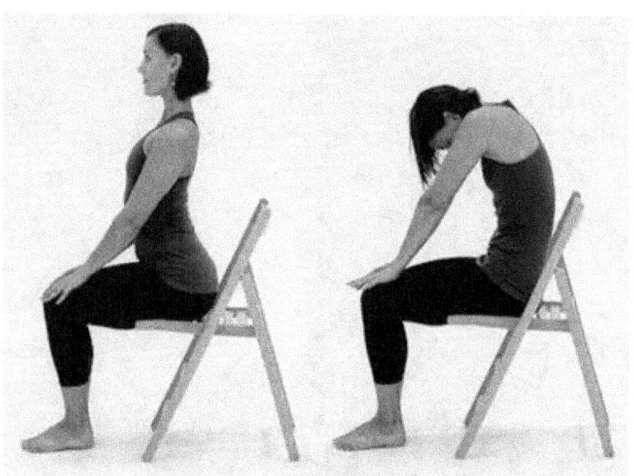

- Sit forward in the chair, place hands on knees.

- Inhale, arch your back (Cow), exhale, round your spine (Cat).

Day 3: *Seated Forward Fold*

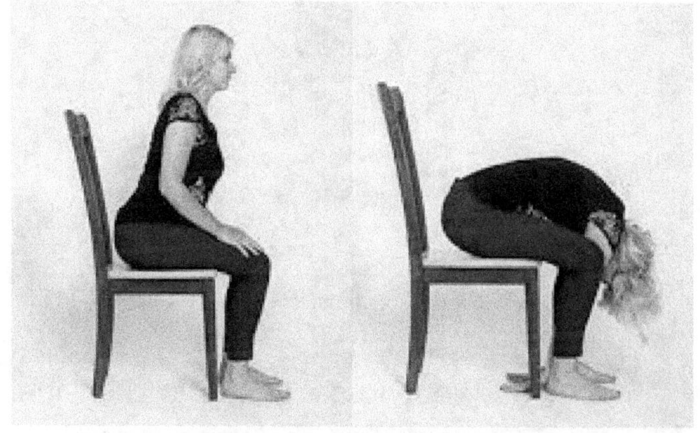

- Sit on the edge of the chair, feet hip-width apart.

- Hinge at the hips, slowly fold forward, reaching for your feet or shins.

Day 4: *Seated Spinal Twist*

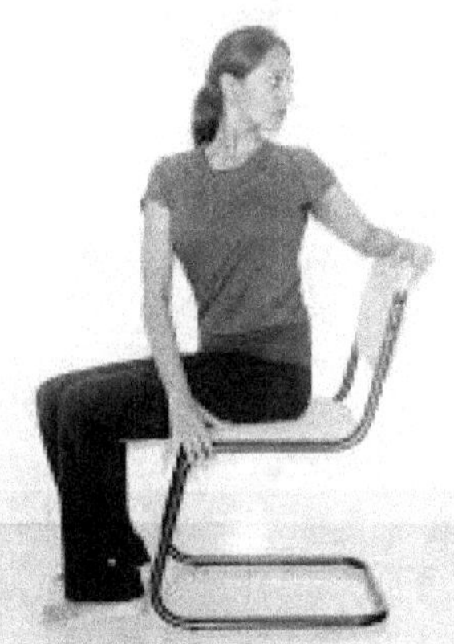

- Sit tall, cross one leg over the other.

- Twist your torso gently to the side, using the chair's back for support.

ENHANCE MOBILITY

Day 5: *Seated Side Stretch*

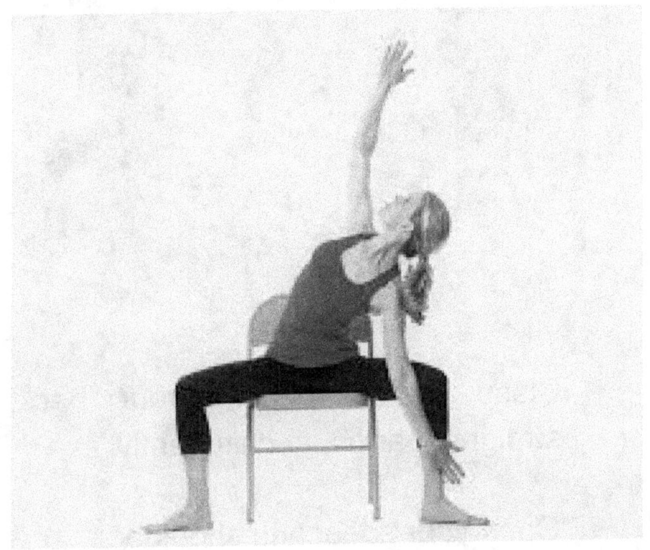

- Sit tall, reach one arm overhead, lean to the opposite side.

- Feel the stretch along your side body.

Day 6: *Seated Shoulder Opener*

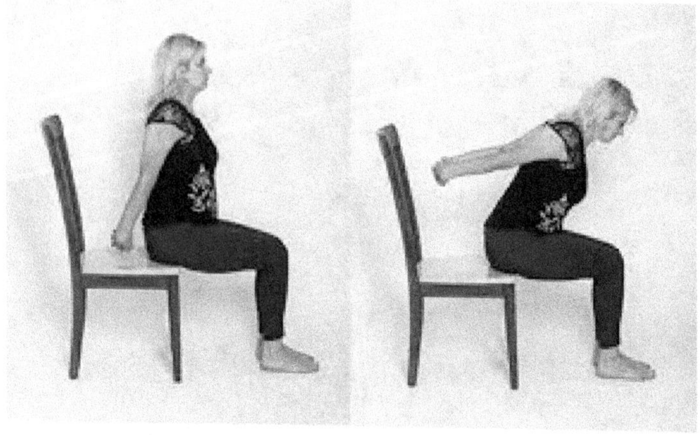

- Clasp hands behind your back, straighten arms, and lift gently.

- Open your chest and shoulders.

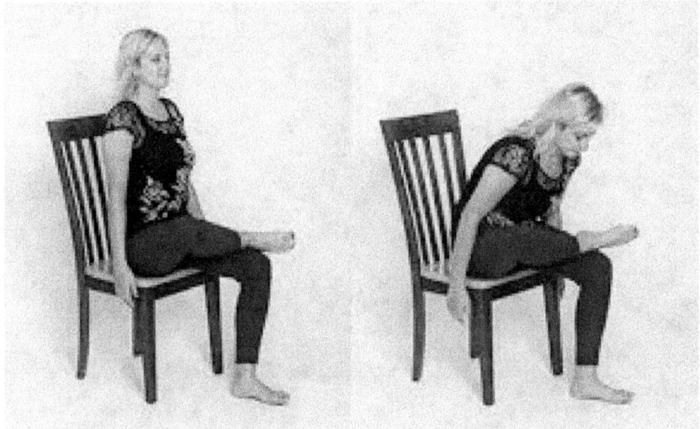

- Sit forward in the chair, cross one ankle over the opposite knee.

- Gently press down on the crossed leg to stretch the hip.

HEART HEALTH AND STAMINATE

Day 8: *Seated Chest Opener*

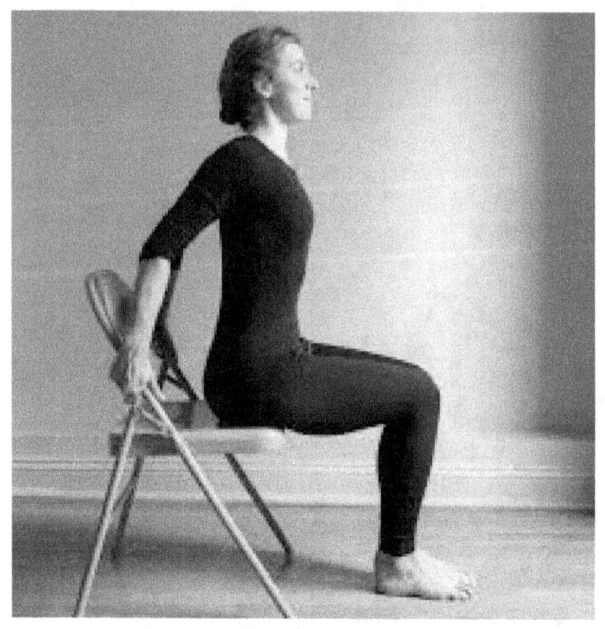

- Sit tall, clasp hands behind your back, straighten arms, and lift while opening the chest.

Day 9: *Seated Warrior Pose*

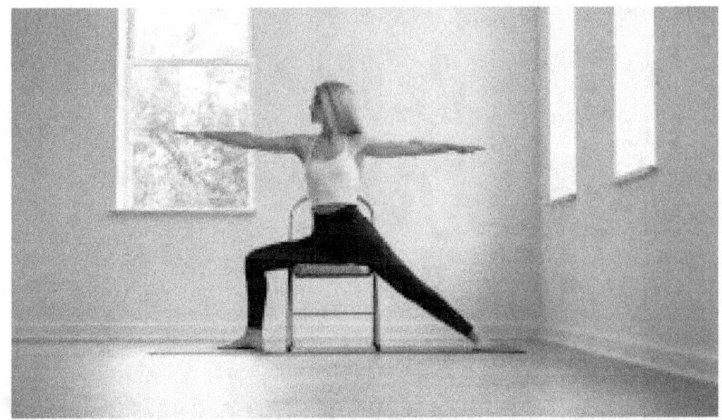

- Sit forward in the chair, extend one leg back, keeping the foot on the ground.

- Lift your arms overhead, feeling a stretch through the torso.

Day 10: *Seated High Lunge*

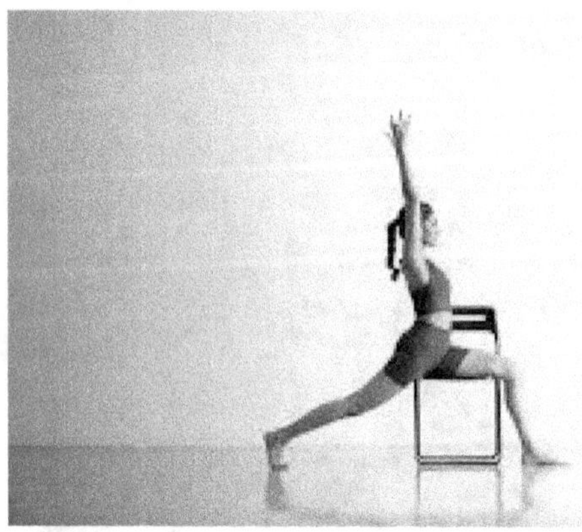

- Sit on the edge of the chair, step one foot back, keeping it on the ground.

- Lift your arms overhead, engaging core muscles.

Day 11: Seated Sun Salutation

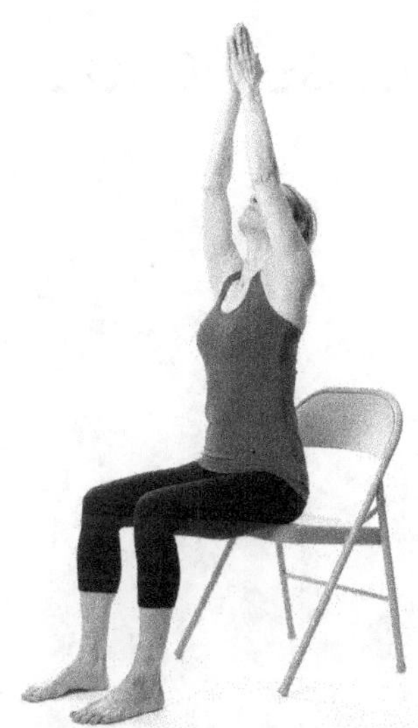

- Flow through a sequence of poses: Seated Mountain, Forward Fold, Seated Cat-Cow, and Seated Upward Stretch.

WEIGHT LOSS FOCUS

Day 12: Seated Knee to Chest

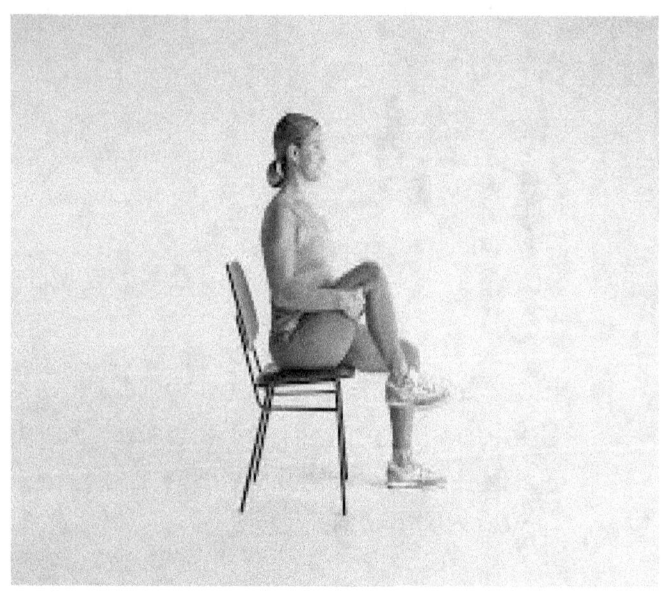

- Sit forward in the chair, hug one knee into your chest.

- Alternate between legs, focusing on controlled breathing.

Day 13: Seated Bicycle Crunches

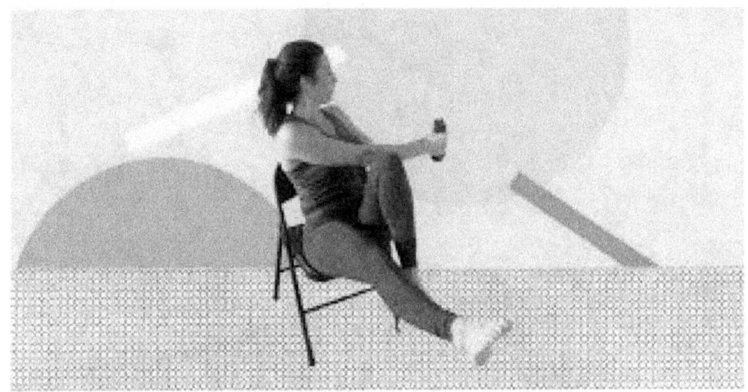

- Sit tall, lean back slightly, lift feet off the ground.

- Mimic cycling motions with your legs, engaging core muscles.

Day 14: Seated Chair Pose

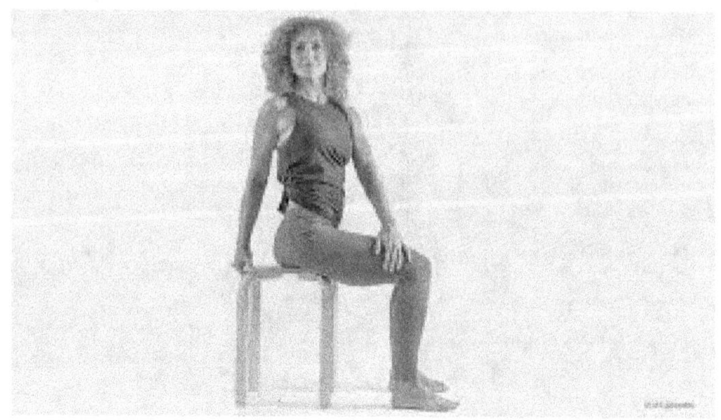

- Sit tall, feet flat on the ground.

- Lean forward slightly, engaging leg muscles as if you're about to stand from the chair.

Continue rotating through these poses, gradually increasing hold times or repetitions as your comfort and capability improve. Always prioritize breath awareness and safety. Adjustments can be made for personal comfort and any physical limitations you may have. Remember, consistency and gradual progress are key in yoga practice!.

CHAPTER 5 CHAIR YOGA AND MEDITATION

BENEFITS OF MEDITATION

Meditation offers a plethora of benefits for both the mind and body. Its advantages extend beyond relaxation and include:

- **Stress Reduction:** By calming the mind, meditation helps reduce stress, which can positively impact overall health.
- **Improved Concentration:** Regular practice enhances focus and attention, which can be beneficial in daily tasks.
- **Emotional Well-being:** It fosters a sense of emotional balance, reducing symptoms of anxiety and depression.
- **Enhanced Self-awareness:** Meditation allows individuals to gain a deeper understanding of themselves, their thoughts, and emotions.
- **Increased Mindfulness:** It cultivates a state of mindfulness, enabling

individuals to live more presently and appreciate each moment.

BASIC MEDITATION POSES FOR BEGINNERS

Chair-based meditation poses cater to beginners who might find sitting on the floor challenging. Some beginner-friendly poses include:

- **Seated Meditation:** Sit comfortably in a chair with feet flat on the ground, hands resting on thighs or in a comfortable position, and focus on the breath.
- **Body Scan:** Start at the top of the head and gradually move focus down through the body, paying attention to sensations and releasing tension.
- **Mindful Breathing:**Focus solely on the breath, noticing the inhales and exhales without trying to change them.

ADVANCED MEDITATION TECHNIQUES

As practitioners progress, they can explore more advanced chair-based meditation techniques such as:

- **Visualization**: Guided imagery meditation, where one imagines serene scenes or peaceful environments, promoting relaxation.
- **Mantra Meditation:** Repeating a word, phrase, or sound silently or aloud, allowing the mind to focus and find tranquility.
- **Loving-KindnessMeditation**: Cultivating feelings of love, compassion, and goodwill towards oneself and others.

TIPS FOR INCORPORATING MEDITATION INTO DAILY LIVING

To integrate meditation into daily life effectively, consider these tips:

- **Consistency**: Set aside a specific time each day for meditation to establish a routine.
- **Start Small:** Begin with short sessions, gradually increasing duration as comfort and confidence grow.
- **Create a Space:** Designate a quiet, comfortable area for meditation to minimize distractions.
- **Be Patient:** Understand that meditation is a practice; progress may take time, and it's okay to have moments of distraction.

By embracing meditation as a part of daily life, individuals can experience profound shifts in their mental, emotional, and physical well-being, all within the ease of a chair-based practice.

CONCLUSION

In drawing our journey to a close within "Chair Yoga for Seniors Over 60," we've explored a path that transcends mere physical exercise. It's been a voyage into the realms of holistic well-being melding the gentle, accessible nature of chair yoga with the serene practice of meditation, tailored specifically for the needs of seniors.

Throughout these pages, we've unfurled the manifold benefits of chair yoga, guiding toward improved flexibility, strength, and mobility, all within the comfort of a seated practice. From postures nurturing posture correction and enhancing mobility to those fostering heart health and aiding weight management, each chapter has aimed to empower and revitalize.

The incorporation of meditation, a cornerstone of this journey, brings forth mindfulness, stress alleviation, and deeper self-awareness. Whether through foundational practices or advanced techniques, these meditative tools open doorways to inner peace and emotional resilience.

Yet, beyond the mere consumption of information lies the heart of this journey to embody and integrate these practices into daily life. It's a commitment not only to physical movement or mental exercises but a pledge to self-care, a promise to honor the temple that is your body and mind.

I encourage you, dear reader, to not just read these words but to live them. Embrace these teachings, weave them into your routine, and let them infuse your days with serenity and strength. May each breath in your chair yoga practice give you vitality, and may each moment in meditation offer tranquility and self-discovery.

May this book become your guiding light, a companion on your voyage to well-being. The true essence lies not in the pages but in the embodiment of these practices. Embrace this journey, and let its transformative power unfurl within you.

Your path to wellness and peace awaits your embrace.

www.ingramcontent.com/pod-product-compliance
Lightning Source LLC
Chambersburg PA
CBHW060846260726
48661CB00002B/631